Ayurvedic Diet Easy Guide for Beginners

Understanding the Importance of Ayurvedic Diet

By

Duthac Garvie

Copyright@2023

Table of Contents

CHAPTER 1

Introduction

1.1 What is Ayurveda?

Ayurveda is an ancient holistic system of medicine that has been practiced for over 5,000 years in the Indian subcontinent. The term "Ayurveda" is derived from two Sanskrit words: "Ayur," meaning life, and "Veda," meaning knowledge or science. This system of medicine is often referred to as the "Science of Life" or the "Art of Living" because it encompasses a comprehensive approach to health and well-being.

At its core, Ayurveda seeks to balance the physical, mental, and spiritual aspects of an individual's life. It is based on the fundamental belief that every person is unique and has a distinct constitution or "Prakriti." This constitution is determined by the balance of three fundamental energies or doshas: Vata, Pitta, and Kapha.

The doshas represent different combinations of the five elements (earth, water, fire, air, and ether) and influence various physiological and psychological aspects of a person's life. Vata is associated with air and ether, Pitta with fire and water, and Kapha with earth and water. By understanding one's dosha and constitution, Ayurveda provides insights into one's natural tendencies, strengths, and weaknesses.

Ayurveda encompasses a wide range of practices, including diet, herbal medicine, yoga, meditation, and lifestyle recommendations. It places a strong emphasis on the prevention of diseases and the promotion of longevity by harmonizing the doshas and maintaining a state of balance in the body and mind.

1.2 The Importance of Ayurvedic Diet

The Ayurvedic diet is a fundamental aspect of Ayurvedic medicine, and it plays a pivotal role in maintaining health, preventing illness, and promoting overall well-being. In Ayurveda, food is not merely a source of sustenance but is considered a powerful tool for healing and maintaining balance in the body.

Here are several key points highlighting the importance of the Ayurvedic diet:

1. **Personalized Nutrition:** One of the core principles of Ayurveda is recognizing that every individual is unique. The Ayurvedic diet takes into account an individual's constitution (Prakriti) and their current imbalances (Vikriti) to create a personalized nutrition plan. This means that what works for one person may not work for another, as their dietary needs are different.

2. **Balancing the Doshas:** Ayurvedic dietary guidelines are tailored to help balance the doshas. For example, if someone has an excess of Pitta energy, they may be

recommended cooling and soothing foods to pacify it. If Vata is predominant, they might need grounding and nourishing foods. Balancing the doshas through diet is seen as a key way to prevent disease and maintain health.

3. **Emphasis on Whole Foods:** Ayurvedic diets prioritize whole, unprocessed foods. Fresh fruits and vegetables, whole grains, legumes, and lean proteins are often recommended. Avoiding processed and artificial foods helps maintain vitality and supports overall health.

4. **Seasonal Eating:** Ayurveda recognizes that the body's needs change with the seasons. Eating seasonal, locally sourced foods

is considered important to stay in harmony with nature and maintain balance. For example, in summer, cooling foods are recommended, while in winter, warming foods are favored.

5. **Digestive Health:** Ayurveda places great emphasis on the strength of one's digestive fire, known as "Agni." A strong Agni is crucial for proper digestion and absorption of nutrients. The Ayurvedic diet offers strategies for enhancing Agni, such as eating at regular times, consuming appropriate foods for one's constitution, and practicing mindful eating.

6. **Mind-Body Connection:** Ayurveda recognizes the profound connection between the mind and the body. The diet

is not only about physical nourishment but also about nurturing emotional and mental well-being. It promotes mindful eating, where individuals are encouraged to savor their food and eat with gratitude and awareness.

Ayurvedic diet is a cornerstone of Ayurvedic medicine, with its focus on personalized nutrition, dosha balancing, and holistic well-being. It recognizes the intimate connection between what we eat and our physical, mental, and spiritual health, making it a valuable system for those seeking a balanced and harmonious way of life.

CHAPTER 2

Ayurvedic Principles

2.1 Understanding the Doshas

In Ayurveda, understanding the doshas is fundamental to maintaining physical and mental health. The doshas are three essential energies or bio-elements that govern various bodily and psychological functions. They are Vata, Pitta, and Kapha, each of which is associated with specific qualities and elements:

- **Vata:** Vata is associated with the elements of air and ether. It embodies qualities such as dryness, lightness, coldness, mobility, and change. Vata governs functions related to movement, including breathing, circulation, and communication. When in balance, Vata individuals are creative, enthusiastic, and agile. However, an excess of Vata can lead to anxiety, restlessness, and digestive issues.

- **Pitta:** Pitta is connected to the elements of fire and water. It represents qualities like heat, sharpness, intensity, and transformation. Pitta regulates digestion, metabolism, and body temperature. Balanced Pitta individuals are intelligent, organized, and have strong digestion. When Pitta is in excess, it can lead to irritability, inflammation, and digestive problems.

- **Kapha:** Kapha relates to the elements of earth and water. Its qualities include heaviness, coldness, stability, and lubrication. Kapha is responsible for structure, stability, and growth. Balanced Kapha individuals are calm, compassionate, and have strong immunity. Excessive Kapha may manifest as lethargy, weight gain, and congestion.

Understanding your dominant dosha and any imbalances is crucial in Ayurveda. Your constitution, known as "Prakriti," is the unique combination of these doshas you are born with, which largely remains constant throughout your life.

Identifying your Prakriti allows you to make informed dietary and lifestyle choices that support your inherent nature.

2.2 The Five Elements in Ayurveda

Ayurveda is deeply rooted in the concept of the five elements, which are the building blocks of the universe and the human body. These elements are:

- **Earth (Prithvi):** Represents solidity, stability, and structure. It is associated with bones, muscles, and tissues in the body.

- **Water (Jala):** Symbolizes fluidity, cohesion, and adaptability. It corresponds to bodily fluids and processes like circulation.

- **Fire (Agni):** Signifies transformation, energy, and metabolism. It governs digestion and the production of energy.

- **Air (Vayu):** Reflects movement, lightness, and mobility. It influences breathing, circulation, and neurological functions.

- **Ether (Akasha):** Represents space and expansiveness. It relates to consciousness, the subtle energy that connects all things.

These elements combine to form the doshas, and their qualities help us understand how various substances and energies interact within the body and the environment. Ayurveda teaches that an individual's constitution and imbalances can be influenced by the interplay of these elements.

2.3 Prakriti and Vikriti: Your Unique Constitution

In Ayurveda, "Prakriti" and "Vikriti" are two fundamental concepts that guide the understanding of an individual's health and well-being.

- **Prakriti:** Prakriti refers to your inherent, genetic constitution. It is the unique combination of the doshas that you are born with and remains relatively stable throughout your life. Knowing your Prakriti allows you to make choices that align with your natural tendencies and maintain a state of balance.

- **Vikriti:** Vikriti, on the other hand, represents your current state of imbalances or deviations from your Prakriti. It is the result of environmental factors, lifestyle choices, and other influences that have affected your doshic balance. Understanding your Vikriti helps Ayurvedic practitioners identify the root causes of health issues and provides a roadmap for bringing the doshas back into equilibrium.

The relationship between Prakriti and Vikriti is central to Ayurvedic diagnosis and treatment. By recognizing your unique constitution and addressing any imbalances, you can optimize your health and well-being by tailoring your diet, lifestyle, and therapeutic interventions to your individual needs. This personalized approach is a hallmark of Ayurveda and is key to achieving and maintaining good health.

CHAPTER 3
The Three Doshas

3.1 Vata Dosha

Characteristics and Traits

Vata is one of the three primary doshas in Ayurveda, and it is associated with the elements of air and ether (space). Vata is characterized by specific qualities and traits:

- **Qualities:**

    - **Dry:** Vata is dry in nature, which can

manifest as dry skin, hair, and a tendency toward constipation.

- **Light:** Vata is lightweight, which can lead to a tendency for individuals with dominant Vata to be underweight.

- **Cold:** Vata is cold, resulting in a low tolerance for cold weather and a preference for warmth.

- **Rough:** Vata can make the skin and hair coarse and prone to roughness.

- **Mobile:** Vata is highly mobile, both in the body and mind, leading to restlessness and rapid thinking.

- **Traits:**

  - Vata individuals are often creative, imaginative, and quick thinkers.

  - They are prone to anxiety, nervousness, and irregular sleep patterns.

  - Vata types have variable appetites and digestion, which can lead to fluctuations in hunger and energy levels.

  - They tend to be adaptable and flexible but may struggle with consistency.

Balancing Vata

Balancing Vata is essential for maintaining health and well-being. Here are some strategies to balance excessive Vata:

- **Diet:** Vata types benefit from warm, nourishing, and grounding foods. This includes cooked grains, root vegetables, and warming spices like ginger and cinnamon. They should avoid cold, raw foods and excessive caffeine.

- **Lifestyle:** Regular routines and warm oil massages (abhyanga) can help soothe Vata. Adequate rest and a calming environment are crucial.

- **Yoga and Exercise:** Gentle, grounding exercises like hatha yoga and tai chi are ideal for Vata. They should avoid overly intense or erratic physical activities.

- **Mindfulness:** Vata individuals can benefit from mindfulness practices that help calm their restless minds, such as meditation and deep breathing exercises.

3.2 Pitta Dosha

Characteristics and Traits

Pitta is the dosha associated with the elements of fire and water. It embodies specific qualities and traits:

- **Qualities:**

  - **Hot:** Pitta is characterized by heat, which can manifest as a

strong metabolism and a
tendency to feel warm,
both in body temperature
and temperament.

- **Sharp:** Pitta is sharp,
leading to a keen intellect
and strong digestion.

- **Light:** Pitta individuals
may have a moderate
build and a preference
for light and cooling
foods.

- **Oily:** Pitta is oily, which
can result in healthy,
lustrous skin but also
make them prone to acne
and oil-related skin
issues.

- **Liquid:** The water
element in Pitta leads to

balanced hydration and fluid balance.

- **Traits:**

  - Pitta types are often ambitious, confident, and have strong leadership qualities.

  - They can be competitive and perfectionistic, and their fiery nature may lead to irritability and anger when imbalanced.

  - They have a strong appetite and efficient digestion.

  - Pitta individuals tend to be organized and structured in their approach to life.

Balancing Pitta

Balancing Pitta is crucial to prevent imbalances and maintain health. Here are some strategies to balance excessive Pitta:

- **Diet:** Pitta types benefit from cooling, hydrating foods such as fresh fruits, vegetables, and dairy. They should avoid spicy and excessively hot foods.

- **Lifestyle:** Pitta individuals should aim for a balanced routine with adequate rest. Avoiding overheating and stressful situations is essential.

- **Yoga and Exercise:** Cooling, calming practices like yin yoga or swimming can help balance Pitta. Avoid excessive heat and strenuous workouts.

- **Mindfulness:** Pitta individuals can benefit from relaxation techniques, such as meditation and progressive muscle relaxation, to manage their intensity and temper.

Understanding and balancing your dominant dosha, whether it's Vata or Pitta, is key to maintaining your physical and mental well-being according to Ayurvedic principles. Balancing these doshas can help you live a healthier and more harmonious life.

3.3 Kapha Dosha

Characteristics and Traits

Kapha is one of the three primary doshas in Ayurveda, and it is associated with the elements of earth and water. Kapha embodies specific qualities and traits:

- **Qualities:**

    - **Heavy:** Kapha is characterized by its heaviness, which can lead to a tendency for individuals with dominant Kapha to gain weight and feel lethargic.

    - **Cold:** Kapha is cold, making Kapha types less tolerant of cold weather and more prone to feeling chilled.

    - **Oily:** Kapha is oily in nature, which can result in soft, smooth skin but may also lead to issues like oily hair and congestion.

- **Stable:** Kapha is stable and solid, which can manifest as a sturdy build and a strong immune system.

- **Moist:** The water element in Kapha leads to balanced hydration and nourishment.

- **Traits:**

  - Kapha individuals are often calm, patient, and compassionate.

  - They have a steady and reliable nature but may be resistant to change.

  - Kapha types tend to be nurturing and enjoy taking care of others.

- They have a consistent appetite and digestion, and they may be prone to cravings for sweet and heavy foods.

Balancing Kapha

Balancing Kapha is essential for maintaining health and well-being. Here are some strategies to balance excessive Kapha:

- **Diet:** Kapha types benefit from warm, light, and stimulating foods. This includes spices like ginger and black pepper and a preference for pungent, bitter, and astringent tastes. They should avoid heavy, oily, and sweet foods.

- **Lifestyle:** Kapha individuals should incorporate regular exercise and movement into their daily routine. Avoiding excessive sleep and creating a dynamic, active lifestyle is important.

- **Yoga and Exercise:** Vigorous, stimulating exercises like aerobics, jogging, or high-intensity interval training can help balance Kapha. Regular physical activity is crucial.

- **Mindfulness:** Kapha individuals may benefit from activities that stimulate the mind and emotions, such as engaging in creative pursuits or practicing invigorating forms of meditation.

Balancing your dominant dosha, whether it's Vata, Pitta, or Kapha, is essential for maintaining physical and mental well-being according to

Ayurvedic principles. Balancing Kapha involves making lifestyle and dietary choices that counteract the qualities and traits associated with excess Kapha, ultimately promoting vitality, energy, and overall health.

CHAPTER 4

Ayurvedic Diet Fundamentals

4.1 The Six Tastes (Rasas)

In Ayurveda, the concept of "Rasas" refers to the six tastes that are essential in an Ayurvedic diet. Each taste has a specific influence on the doshas and can either balance or aggravate them. The six tastes are:

1. **Sweet (Madhura):** Sweet taste is associated with the earth and water elements. It has a grounding and nourishing quality and can pacify Vata and

Pitta doshas. Foods like grains, legumes, and naturally sweet fruits fall into this category.

2. **Sour (Amla):** The sour taste is linked to the fire and earth elements. It can stimulate digestion and balance Vata but can aggravate Pitta and Kapha. Sour foods include citrus fruits, yogurt, and vinegar.

3. **Salty (Lavana):** Saltiness corresponds to the water and fire elements. It can pacify Vata and add flavor to dishes, but excessive salt intake can aggravate Pitta and Kapha. Salty foods include sea salt, seaweed, and certain vegetables.

4. **Bitter (Tikta):** Bitter taste is associated with the air and ether

elements. It is cooling and detoxifying and helps balance Pitta and Kapha but may increase Vata. Bitter foods include dark leafy greens, turmeric, and bitter melon.

5. **Pungent (Katu):** Pungent taste is related to the fire and air elements. It can stimulate digestion, clear congestion, and balance Kapha, but it can aggravate Pitta and Vata. Pungent foods include chili peppers, garlic, and mustard.

6. **Astringent (Kashaya):** The astringent taste is linked to the earth and air elements. It has a drying and cooling quality and can balance Pitta and Kapha while potentially aggravating Vata. Astringent foods include

legumes, green bananas, and certain beans.

The balance of these tastes in your diet is crucial to maintain harmony and prevent imbalances of the doshas. Ayurvedic practitioners often recommend tailoring your meals to include all six tastes in each meal, with an emphasis on the tastes that help balance your specific constitution and current state (Vikriti).

4.2 Seasonal Eating

Ayurveda emphasizes the importance of eating seasonally to maintain balance and health. Each season is associated with different qualities and doshic influences. Here are some key principles of seasonal eating in Ayurveda:

- **Spring (March to May):** Spring is a Kapha-increasing season. To balance this, favor foods that are lighter, drier, and slightly spicy to reduce Kapha's heaviness and congestion.

- **Summer (June to August):** Summer is characterized by increased Pitta energy. Choose foods that are cooling, hydrating, and slightly bitter or astringent to pacify Pitta's heat.

- **Autumn (September to November):** Autumn is a Vata-predominant season. Opt for warm, grounding, and nourishing foods to counterbalance Vata's dryness and instability.

- **Winter (December to February):** Winter is also a

Kapha-increasing season. Focus on warm, hearty, and slightly spicy foods to counteract Kapha's cold and damp tendencies.

Eating seasonally aligns your diet with the natural rhythms of the environment, which can help prevent imbalances and support overall well-being.

4.3 Food Combinations

Ayurveda provides guidelines for combining foods to optimize digestion and nutrient absorption. Proper food combinations can reduce digestive discomfort and promote better assimilation of nutrients. Some general principles include:

- **Avoid combining milk with sour, salty, or heat-producing foods.**

- **Do not combine fruits with dairy or grains.**

- **Limit combining proteins (e.g., meat, dairy, legumes) with carbohydrates (e.g., grains or starchy vegetables).**

- **Include spices like ginger and cumin to aid digestion.**

These guidelines are intended to maintain the digestive fire (Agni) and prevent the formation of Ama, a toxic substance that can lead to various health issues.

4.4 Cooking Methods

Ayurveda also places importance on the way food is prepared and cooked. Different cooking methods can influence the qualities of the food and its impact on the doshas. Here are some key cooking methods and their doshic effects:

- **Boiling:** Boiling is seen as a balancing method that can pacify all three doshas. It is especially beneficial for Vata types.

- **Roasting:** Roasting can balance Vata and Kapha but may aggravate Pitta. It is a heating method and can dry out food.

- **Steaming:** Steaming is a balanced method that can pacify all doshas. It helps retain the food's moisture and nutrients.

- **Sautéing:** Sautéing with ghee or oil can balance Vata and Kapha but may aggravate Pitta due to the heat.

- **Frying:** Deep frying is heating and can aggravate all doshas, especially Pitta. It is not commonly recommended in Ayurveda.

By understanding the doshic effects of various cooking methods, you can tailor your meal preparation to your constitution and current imbalances, promoting better digestion and overall well-being.

CHAPTER 5

Ayurvedic Food Choices

5.1 Vata-Pacifying Foods

Vata-pacifying foods are essential for balancing the Vata dosha, which is characterized by qualities like cold, dry, light, and mobile. To soothe Vata and maintain balance, it's important to include foods that have opposite qualities. Here are some examples of Vata-pacifying foods:

- **Sweet Fruits:** Sweet, ripe fruits like bananas, avocados, mangoes, and melons provide nourishment and help balance Vata's dryness.

- **Cooked Vegetables:** Cooked, warm, and well-cooked vegetables like sweet potatoes, carrots, and beets are grounding and easy to digest.

- **Nuts and Seeds:** Soaked and lightly roasted nuts and seeds like almonds, sesame seeds, and flaxseeds can provide healthy fats and warmth.

- **Grains:** Nourishing grains like rice, oats, and quinoa are Vata-pacifying, especially when cooked with ghee or oil.

- **Legumes:** Well-cooked lentils, mung beans, and split peas are good protein sources for Vata individuals.

- **Dairy:** Warm, whole dairy products like milk, ghee, and yogurt can be included in moderation to support Vata.

- **Spices:** Vata types benefit from warming spices like ginger, cinnamon, and cumin to aid digestion.

- **Herbal Teas:** Warm, herbal teas like ginger tea or cinnamon tea can help balance Vata.

5.2 Pitta-Pacifying Foods

Pitta-pacifying foods are essential for balancing the Pitta dosha, which is characterized by qualities like heat, sharpness, and intensity. To cool and soothe Pitta, it's important to include foods that have opposite qualities. Here are some examples of Pitta-pacifying foods:

- **Sweet Fruits:** Sweet, ripe fruits like melons, pears, and sweet apples can help cool down Pitta's heat.

- **Bitter Vegetables:** Bitter vegetables like leafy greens, bitter melon, and zucchini have a cooling effect on Pitta.

- **Dairy:** Cooling dairy products like milk, coconut milk, and unsalted butter can be included in moderation.

- **Grains:** Soothing grains like basmati rice, barley, and oats provide a stable source of energy.

- **Legumes:** Mung beans and tofu are excellent protein sources for Pitta types.

- **Cooling Oils:** Coconut oil and sunflower oil can be used for cooking, as they have a cooling effect.

- **Spices:** Mild, cooling spices like coriander, fennel, and cardamom can be used to flavor dishes.

- **Herbal Teas:** Herbal teas with peppermint, chamomile, or licorice root can help cool down Pitta and aid digestion.

It's important to note that these food choices should be tailored to your individual constitution and any current imbalances (Vikriti). While these guidelines provide a general framework, a personalized approach, ideally under the guidance of an Ayurvedic practitioner, is best for optimal results.

5.3 Kapha-Pacifying Foods

Kapha-pacifying foods are crucial for balancing the Kapha dosha, which is characterized by qualities like heaviness, coldness, and stability. To counterbalance Kapha's tendencies, it's important to incorporate foods that have opposite qualities. Here are some examples of Kapha-pacifying foods:

- **Bitter Greens:** Bitter leafy greens like kale, collard greens, and dandelion greens help to reduce excess Kapha by promoting digestion and detoxification.

- **Astringent Fruits:** Astringent fruits like apples, pomegranates, and cranberries can help balance Kapha by reducing excess moisture and mucus.

- **Legumes:** Light and easily digestible legumes such as lentils and mung beans are good protein sources for Kapha types.

- **Grains:** Light grains like millet and quinoa are suitable for Kapha, as they are less likely to promote heaviness.

- **Pungent Vegetables:** Pungent vegetables like radishes, mustard greens, and daikon radishes can help stimulate digestion and reduce congestion.

- **Spices:** Warming and pungent spices like ginger, black pepper, and cayenne can aid digestion and balance Kapha.

- **Herbal Teas:** Herbal teas with ginger, cinnamon, and cloves can help warm and invigorate Kapha.

- **Honey:** In moderation, honey can be a sweetener for Kapha, as long as it's not too heavy or cold.

- **Light Proteins:** Light proteins such as fish and poultry can be included in moderation for Kapha individuals.

It's essential to customize your food choices to align with your individual constitution and any current imbalances (Vikriti). While these guidelines provide a general framework, a personalized approach, ideally under the guidance of an Ayurvedic practitioner, is the best way to achieve optimal results. Balancing your doshas through diet can help maintain overall well-being and prevent health issues associated with doshic imbalances.

CHAPTER 6

Meal Planning

6.1 Designing Balanced Meals

Designing balanced meals in Ayurveda is essential to ensure that your diet supports your unique constitution and promotes overall well-being. A balanced meal typically includes all six tastes (sweet, sour, salty, bitter, pungent, and astringent) in proportions that are appropriate for your dosha. Here are some general principles for designing balanced meals in Ayurveda:

- **Include a variety of foods:** A balanced meal should include a diverse range of whole, fresh foods, including grains, legumes, vegetables, and a source of protein.

- **Choose seasonal and local ingredients:** Eating foods that are in season and sourced locally aligns your diet with the rhythms of nature and helps maintain balance.

- **Adjust portion sizes:** Portion sizes should be adjusted to your individual constitution and current state (Prakriti and Vikriti). Vata types may need smaller, more frequent meals, while Kapha types may require smaller portions to prevent overeating.

- **Mindful eating:** Pay attention to the quality of your food, your state of mind while eating, and the way you chew and digest your food. Mindful eating promotes better digestion and absorption.

- **Hydration:** Sip warm water or herbal teas with your meals, as cold drinks can weaken digestion. Avoid drinking too much during meals to prevent diluting digestive juices.

- **Opt for freshly prepared meals:** Freshly cooked meals are preferred over leftovers or packaged foods to ensure the highest nutritional value and prana (life force).

6.2 Ayurvedic Breakfast Ideas

Breakfast is considered an important meal in Ayurveda, and it should be nourishing and suited to your dosha. Here are some Ayurvedic breakfast ideas for each dosha:

- **Vata Breakfast:**

    - Cream of rice or oatmeal with warm milk and a pinch of cardamom and nutmeg.

    - A fruit smoothie with ripe banana, dates, almond milk, and a touch of ghee.

    - Whole-grain toast with almond butter and honey.

- **Pitta Breakfast:**

- Cooled, cooked grains like quinoa with fresh berries and a drizzle of honey.

- A fruit salad with sweet, cooling fruits like melons, and a sprinkle of mint.

- Greek yogurt with sliced cucumber and a dash of fresh cilantro.

- **Kapha Breakfast:**

  - Warm, spiced oatmeal with chopped apples and a sprinkle of cinnamon.

  - Lightly toasted whole-grain bread with a small amount of ghee and a slice of orange.

- Scrambled eggs with sautéed asparagus and a pinch of black pepper.

6.3 Ayurvedic Lunch Ideas

Lunch is typically the largest meal of the day in Ayurveda, as it coincides with the peak of digestive fire (Agni). Here are some Ayurvedic lunch ideas:

- **Vata Lunch:**

  - Basmati rice with mung dal (lentils), steamed vegetables, and a dollop of ghee.

  - A mixed vegetable soup with warming spices like cumin and ginger.

- Sweet potato and spinach curry with whole wheat chapati.

- **Pitta Lunch:**

  - Quinoa salad with cucumber, mint, and a lemon-tahini dressing.

  - Stir-fried vegetables with tofu and a cooling cilantro chutney.

  - A lentil and rice dish (khichdi) with a side of yogurt.

- **Kapha Lunch:**

  - Chickpea and vegetable stew with warming spices like turmeric and black pepper.

- A light and spicy tomato soup with a side of mixed greens.

- Steamed broccoli and quinoa with a sprinkle of sesame seeds.

These meal ideas can be adjusted based on your individual constitution and any current imbalances. Ayurvedic meal planning is highly personalized, and consulting with an Ayurvedic practitioner can provide further guidance for your specific needs.

6.4 Ayurvedic Dinner Ideas

Dinner in Ayurveda is generally lighter than lunch and should be eaten at least two hours before bedtime to allow for proper digestion. Here are some Ayurvedic dinner ideas for each dosha:

- **Vata Dinner:**

    - Quinoa or millet with steamed vegetables and a dash of ghee.

    - A light, warming lentil soup with a side of cooked greens.

    - Baked sweet potatoes with a sprinkle of cinnamon.

- **Pitta Dinner:**

    - Vegetable stir-fry with tofu and a cooling coconut milk sauce.

    - Rice with a side of cucumber raita (yogurt

with cucumber and
spices).

- Grilled fish with a side of sautéed zucchini and mint.

- **Kapha Dinner:**

  - Spiced mung bean soup with a hint of ginger and turmeric.

  - Steamed broccoli and carrots with quinoa and a drizzle of lemon juice.

  - Lightly sautéed asparagus with a side of quinoa.

6.5 Snacks and Beverages

In Ayurveda, snacks should be light and easy to digest. Here are some Ayurvedic snack and beverage ideas:

- **Fruit:** Fresh, ripe fruit is an excellent snack. Apples, pears, and berries are often good choices. Avoid eating fruit right after a meal to prevent digestive disturbances.

- **Nuts:** A small handful of soaked and lightly roasted nuts like almonds or walnuts can provide a satisfying snack.

- **Herbal Teas:** Herbal teas like ginger, chamomile, or fennel can be enjoyed between meals. Choose teas that complement your dosha or address specific imbalances.

- **Lassi:** A cooling yogurt-based drink can be made with yogurt, water, and a pinch of cardamom or cumin. Sweeten with a touch of honey for Vata and Pitta or a small amount of rock salt for Kapha.

- **Popcorn:** Lightly seasoned popcorn with ghee and a pinch of your preferred spices can be a satisfying snack when prepared mindfully.

- **Rice Cakes:** Whole grain rice cakes with almond butter or hummus can provide a quick and easy snack.

- **Fresh Vegetable Sticks:** Sliced cucumbers, carrots, or celery with a light dip of hummus or

tahini can be a refreshing
snack.

Remember to eat snacks in moderation and be mindful of your individual constitution and any current imbalances. The key is to choose foods and beverages that support your overall well-being and align with your doshic needs.

CHAPTER 7

Ayurvedic Lifestyle Practices

7.1 Ayurvedic Lifestyle Practices

In Ayurveda, lifestyle practices are considered just as important as diet in maintaining health and preventing imbalances. These practices aim to harmonize the doshas, align your daily routine with the natural rhythms of the day, and foster physical and mental well-being. Here are some key Ayurvedic lifestyle practices:

Daily Routines (Dinacharya)

- **Wake Up Early:** Ideally, rise before sunrise (Brahma muhurta) to synchronize your body with the natural rhythm of the day.

- **Oral Care:** Upon waking, scrape your tongue to remove Ama (toxins), then brush your teeth. You can use herbal toothpaste or a toothpowder.

- **Oil Pulling:** Swish coconut or sesame oil in your mouth for a few minutes to promote oral and systemic health. Spit it out and rinse your mouth afterward.

- **Nasal Cleansing (Neti):** Use a neti pot to clean the nasal passages with saline water, particularly if you have congestion or allergies.

- **Hydration:** Drink a glass of warm water to stimulate digestion and hydrate your body.

- **Bowel Movement:** Attend to the call of nature to ensure a healthy elimination process.

- **Self-Massage (Abhyanga):** Apply warm oil to your body, massaging it in gentle, circular motions. This practice nourishes the skin, calms the mind, and balances the doshas.

- **Bathing:** Take a warm shower or bath to clean the body and refresh the mind.

- **Exercise:** Engage in a form of exercise that aligns with your dosha and constitution. Yoga, tai chi, or a morning walk can be beneficial.

- **Meditation or Mindfulness:** Dedicate time to calm your mind, whether through meditation, deep breathing exercises, or mindfulness practices.

- **Breakfast:** Eat a balanced, nourishing breakfast according to your dosha.

- **Work and Activities:** Plan your day's activities, incorporating breaks to rest and eat. Try to eat your main meal at lunchtime when digestion is strongest.

- **Dinner:** Opt for a lighter, earlier dinner to ensure proper digestion and to avoid heavy, late-night meals.

- **Sleep:** Aim for quality sleep by going to bed early, sleeping in a dark, quiet room, and maintaining a regular sleep schedule.

7.2 Seasonal Routines (Ritucharya)

Ritucharya refers to seasonal routines, which are crucial in Ayurveda for maintaining balance throughout the year. Each season has its unique qualities, and adjusting your lifestyle practices can help prevent imbalances. Here's a general overview:

- **Spring (Vasanta):** As the weather warms up and Kapha tends to accumulate, focus on cleansing practices like detoxification and dietary adjustments.

- **Summer (Grishma):** Pitta energy intensifies in the summer. Stay cool, hydrated, and protect your skin from the sun. Favor cooling foods and drinks.

- **Monsoon (Varsha):** During the monsoon season, Kapha can be aggravated. Focus on digestive health and consider detoxification practices.

- **Autumn (Sharad):** As Vata energy increases, it's important to establish routines that promote stability, nourishment, and grounding.

- **Late Autumn (Hemanta):** Similar to autumn, address Vata imbalances and focus on nourishing, warm, and moistening practices.

- **Winter (Shishira):** Pitta and Kapha imbalances can occur in the winter. Stay warm, eat nourishing foods, and engage in warming practices.

Adapting your lifestyle practices to the changing seasons helps harmonize your body with the external environment and supports your overall health and well-being in accordance with Ayurvedic principles.

7.3 Yoga and Exercise

Yoga and exercise play a crucial role in Ayurvedic lifestyle practices, promoting physical health, mental well-being, and balance among the doshas. The choice of yoga and exercise should be tailored to your constitution and any current imbalances. Here are some key principles related to yoga and exercise in Ayurveda:

- **Yoga:** Yoga is a holistic practice that encompasses physical postures (asanas), breath control (pranayama), meditation, and philosophical principles. The specific type of yoga and asanas you choose should align with your dosha. For example, Vata types may benefit from gentle, grounding practices, while Pitta types might find relief through cooling and calming poses. Kapha types can benefit from more dynamic, invigorating yoga.

- **Exercise:** Regular physical activity is essential for overall health. The type and intensity of exercise should be chosen according to your dosha. Vata types may benefit from gentle forms of exercise, while Pitta individuals can engage in moderate activities, and Kapha types may need more vigorous exercise to combat sluggishness.

- **Balance:** Balance is a key concept in Ayurvedic exercise. Overexercising can lead to the aggravation of doshas, while underexercising can contribute to imbalances. It's essential to strike a balance that supports your constitution and current state.

- **Seasonal Variation:** Adjust your exercise routine based on the season. In colder seasons, Vata and Kapha types may need to increase their activity levels, while Pitta individuals might benefit from cooling exercises like swimming.

- **Listen to Your Body:** Pay attention to how your body responds to different forms of exercise. Adjust your routine if you experience discomfort or fatigue.

- **Warm-Up and Cool-Down:** Proper warm-up and cool-down routines are crucial to prevent injuries and maintain balance. A brief self-massage with warm oil before exercise can help.

7.4 Stress Management and Mindfulness

Stress management and mindfulness are vital components of an Ayurvedic lifestyle, as they help maintain mental and emotional equilibrium. Stress can disrupt the balance of the doshas and contribute to various health issues. Here are some Ayurvedic strategies for stress management and mindfulness:

- **Meditation:** Regular meditation practices, such as mindfulness meditation (Vipassana), loving-kindness meditation (Metta), or transcendental meditation (TM), can help calm the mind and reduce stress.

- **Deep Breathing:** Incorporate deep breathing exercises, such as pranayama, to reduce stress and improve oxygenation of the body.

- **Yoga Nidra:** Yoga Nidra is a guided relaxation technique that induces deep relaxation and can help alleviate stress and anxiety.

- **Aromatherapy:** The use of essential oils like lavender and rose can have a calming effect and promote relaxation.

- **Mindful Eating:** Pay attention to the quality and quantity of your food, as well as the act of eating itself. Eating mindfully can improve digestion and emotional well-being.

- **Cultivate Positive Emotions:** Practice gratitude, kindness, and positivity to counteract stress and promote emotional balance.

- **Daily Routine:** A structured daily routine (Dinacharya) can help create a sense of stability and predictability, reducing stress.

- **Nature Connection:** Spending time in nature and practicing ecotherapy can be calming and grounding.

- **Limit Screen Time:** Reduce exposure to excessive screen time and electronic devices, especially before bedtime, to support restful sleep and reduce mental stress.

- **Seek Balance:** Balance work, rest, and play in your life to reduce stress and maintain equilibrium.

Stress management and mindfulness practices should be personalized to your dosha and constitution. Regularly incorporating these practices into your daily life can help you manage stress, maintain emotional balance, and support overall well-being according to Ayurvedic principles.

CHAPTER 8

Ayurvedic Remedies and Herbs

8.1 Common Ayurvedic Herbs

Ayurveda relies on a wide range of herbs to maintain health, balance the doshas, and treat various health conditions. Here are some common Ayurvedic herbs and their uses:

- **Ashwagandha (Withania somnifera):** Known as the "Indian ginseng," ashwagandha is an adaptogen that helps the body adapt to stress. It's used to balance Vata and reduce anxiety.

- **Turmeric (Curcuma longa):** A powerful anti-inflammatory and antioxidant, turmeric is used to pacify Pitta and reduce inflammation in the body.

- **Tulsi (Holy Basil):** Tulsi is known for its adaptogenic properties and is used to reduce stress and balance the doshas. It's particularly helpful for Pitta imbalances.

- **Triphala:** This combination of three fruits—amalaki, bibhitaki, and haritaki—supports digestion, detoxification, and balancing all three doshas.

- **Ginger (Zingiber officinale):** Ginger aids digestion, reduces inflammation, and helps balance Kapha.

- **Neem (Azadirachta indica):** Neem is known for its cleansing and detoxifying properties, particularly for skin conditions and imbalances in Pitta and Kapha.

- **Brahmi (Bacopa monnieri):** Brahmi is used to improve cognitive function, reduce stress, and balance Vata and Pitta.

- **Amla (Indian Gooseberry):** Amla is a potent source of vitamin C and is used to boost immunity and reduce excess Pitta.

- **Shatavari (Asparagus racemosus):** Shatavari is a nourishing herb that supports the female reproductive system, balances Vata and Pitta, and cools the body.

- **Guduchi (Tinospora cordifolia):** Guduchi is an immune booster and detoxifier used to reduce fever and balance all three doshas.

- **Haritaki (Terminalia chebula):** Haritaki is one of the three fruits in Triphala and is used to support digestion, detoxification, and Vata balance.

- **Bhringaraj (Eclipta alba)**

- : Bhringaraj is often used for hair health and to reduce excess Pitta.

8.2 Home Remedies for Common Ailments

Ayurveda offers numerous home remedies for common ailments using natural ingredients. Here are some examples:

- **Indigestion:** Mix ginger and lemon juice with a pinch of rock salt and consume to aid digestion.

- **Cough and Cold:** Prepare a tea with honey, ginger, and Tulsi leaves to soothe a sore throat and reduce cough.

- **Constipation:** Consume a ripe banana with a teaspoon of ghee before bedtime to promote regular bowel movements.

- **Headache:** Apply a paste of sandalwood and water on your forehead to relieve headaches.

- **Skin Irritations:** Mix neem powder with water to create a paste and apply it to the affected area to soothe skin irritations.

- **Sore Throat:** Gargle with warm water containing salt, turmeric, and a few drops of ghee to alleviate a sore throat.

- **Stress and Anxiety:** Practice daily meditation and deep breathing exercises to reduce stress and anxiety.

- **Insomnia:** Consume warm milk with a pinch of nutmeg before bedtime to promote restful sleep.

- **Bad Breath:** Chew fennel seeds or cardamom to freshen your breath.

- **Sunburn:** Apply a paste of sandalwood and rosewater to the affected area to soothe sunburn.

These are just a few examples of Ayurvedic home remedies for common ailments. Ayurveda encourages using natural ingredients and practices to address health issues and maintain well-being. Keep in mind that individual constitutions and imbalances may require specific remedies, so it's often beneficial to consult with an Ayurvedic practitioner for personalized guidance

CHAPTER 9

Ayurvedic Diet Challenges

9.1 Ayurvedic Diet Challenges - Overcoming Obstacles

Adopting an Ayurvedic diet and lifestyle can come with its own set of challenges, but with dedication and awareness, you can overcome these obstacles. Here are some common challenges and ways to address them:

Lack of Knowledge: Understanding Ayurvedic principles and guidelines can be a challenge for beginners. To overcome this, consider studying Ayurveda or consulting with an

Ayurvedic practitioner for personalized guidance. There are also many books, websites, and courses available to help you learn more about Ayurveda.

Finding Ayurvedic Ingredients: Some Ayurvedic herbs and ingredients may not be readily available in your local grocery store. Explore international or specialty food markets, or consider purchasing Ayurvedic herbs and spices online.

Balancing Taste Preferences: If your current taste preferences differ from what Ayurveda recommends, it can be challenging to adjust. Gradually introduce Ayurvedic tastes into your diet and explore new recipes to make the transition more enjoyable.

Social and Cultural Factors: Social gatherings and cultural practices often revolve around specific foods. Communicate your dietary needs to friends and family, and seek out Ayurvedic-friendly options when dining out.

Lifestyle Conflicts: Balancing Ayurvedic practices with a busy modern lifestyle can be challenging. Start by incorporating small Ayurvedic rituals into your daily routine, and gradually build on them as you become more comfortable.

Patience and Persistence: Achieving balance and healing through Ayurveda may take time. Be patient and stay persistent, and remember that small changes can have a significant impact on your well-being.

9.2 Adapting to Individual Needs

Ayurveda is highly personalized, and your diet and lifestyle should be adapted to your individual constitution (Prakriti) and current imbalances (Vikriti). Here's how to adapt Ayurvedic practices to your specific needs:

Consult an Ayurvedic Practitioner: To receive personalized guidance, consult with an Ayurvedic practitioner who can assess your constitution, imbalances, and specific health goals. They can create a customized plan that suits your individual needs.

Listen to Your Body: Pay attention to how your body responds to various foods, practices, and lifestyle changes. This self-awareness will help you make adjustments that align with your unique constitution and imbalances.

Seasonal Adaptations: Adjust your diet and lifestyle to the changing seasons. What works for you in one season may need to be adapted in another. For example, a cooling diet may be more suitable in summer, while a warming one may be better in winter.

Flexibility in Approach: Ayurveda provides guidelines, but it's important to be flexible and adapt them to your individual needs. What works for one person may not work for another, and your needs may change over time.

Regular Assessments: Periodically reassess your health and well-being with an Ayurvedic practitioner. As your needs change, so should your Ayurvedic plan.

Adapting Ayurvedic practices to your individual needs is key to experiencing the full benefits of this holistic system of medicine. By addressing your unique constitution and imbalances, you can achieve a state of balance, vitality, and well-being that is tailored to you.

9.3 Embracing Ayurvedic Principles

Embracing Ayurvedic principles is a holistic journey toward wellness that involves aligning your diet, lifestyle, and mindset with the wisdom of Ayurveda. Here are some key steps to help you fully embrace Ayurvedic principles:

Education: Start by learning the fundamentals of Ayurveda. Study the doshas, tastes, and qualities, as well as the principles of Prakriti and Vikriti. This knowledge forms the foundation for Ayurvedic living.

Self-Assessment: Understand your unique constitution (Prakriti) and any current imbalances (Vikriti). This self-assessment is the starting point for tailoring Ayurvedic practices to your individual needs.

Balanced Diet: Begin to incorporate Ayurvedic dietary principles into your meals. Choose foods and spices that align with your dosha and the current season. Gradually reduce or eliminate foods that disrupt your balance.

Lifestyle Practices: Incorporate Ayurvedic lifestyle practices like Dinacharya (daily routines) and Ritucharya (seasonal routines) into your life. These practices help establish balance, promote health, and prevent imbalances.

Mindfulness and Stress Management: Implement mindfulness, meditation, and stress management techniques to foster emotional and mental balance. This includes practices like deep breathing, yoga, and mindful eating.

Consistency: Consistency is key. Establish daily and seasonal routines, and stick to them as closely as possible. This helps your body and mind adapt to Ayurvedic living.

Adaptation: Be open to making adjustments as you learn more about how Ayurveda affects your well-being. Your needs may change over time, and Ayurveda encourages you to adapt to these changes.

9.4 Your Journey to Wellness

Your journey to wellness through Ayurveda is a process that unfolds over time. Here's how you can embark on and navigate this journey:

Setting Intentions: Begin your journey by setting clear intentions for what you hope to achieve with Ayurveda. Whether it's better digestion, stress reduction, or overall well-being, define your goals.

Self-Awareness: Develop self-awareness by paying attention to how your body and mind respond to Ayurvedic practices. Notice the impact of your diet, lifestyle, and mindset on your well-being.

Seek Guidance: If possible, consult with an Ayurvedic practitioner who can provide personalized guidance and support. They can help you make informed choices and adjustments along your journey.

Consistency: Consistency is essential. Embrace Ayurvedic practices on a daily and seasonal basis. While perfection isn't necessary, a commitment to regularity will yield the best results.

Patience: Understand that healing and balance take time. Be patient with yourself and the process. Ayurveda is about gradual, sustainable change.

Flexibility: Be flexible and willing to adapt your Ayurvedic practices as you learn and grow. Your journey is unique, and your needs may evolve over time.

Reflection and Adjustment: Periodically reflect on your journey, assess your progress, and make necessary adjustments. This will help you fine-tune your approach and continue on the path to wellness.

Embracing Ayurvedic principles and embarking on a journey to wellness is a transformative process that can lead to greater physical, mental, and emotional well-being. As you apply these principles and make them a part of your daily life, you'll discover the profound impact of Ayurveda on your overall health and vitality.

www.ingramcontent.com/pod-product-compliance
Lightning Source LLC
Chambersburg PA
CBHW070818280726
48660CB00016B/2124